Farmhouse Classics

Hearty Soups & Broths

Alison Lingard

FARMHOUSE CLASSICS – HEARTY SOUPS & BROTHS

ISBN-13: 978-1-7647445-6-0

Contents

Introduction

Having had the privilege of growing up on a farm I have always cherished those old time classic recipes handed down from generation to generation. The recipes that were a family's best kept secret which often created bickering amongst the siblings over whose was best.

Within this book I have created and collated all those hearty classic soups and broths for your mouth watering pleasure.

Soup is a great way to make the best of seasonal produce. The key to a good soup is allowing enough time for those wholesome herbs and spices to release their flavours in to the broth and meat. Depending on the soup you are making the cooking times can vary from 1 hour to up to 8 hours. The shorter the cook time the more thinner your soup will be and your vegetables will keep more nutrients. The longer the cooking time the more thickly and flavoursome your soup will be. I have tried to cater for both of these desires and everything in between.

One of my favourite memories of these recipes growing up was not only the delicious hearty soups that always left me licking the bowl, but also the toppers or toasted sough dough bread served with the soups. I use to love it when Gran sprinkled her home made croutons over the top, swirled in delicious pesto, yoghurt or cream just before serving or added a sprinkling of freshly chopped chili to warm us up on a cold winter's night. That's the beauty about soups though; the versatility and possibilities are endless! Whether you are making a low cost meal for your family or an exquisite entrée for your dinner guests, I truly hope you enjoy the recipes in this book as much as I have enjoyed making and tweaking them in to quick and simple steps.

Chicken

Lemon Grove Chicken Soup

2 medium chicken breasts, boneless, skinless
6 cloves garlic, peeled and chopped
1 red onion, peeled and chopped.
½ cup egg noodles
2 leeks, chopped
2 lemons, juiced
2 cups low-sodium chicken broth
Extra virgin olive oil

1. Lightly coat 4 qt. slow cooker with olive oil.
2. Cube the chicken.
3. Place chicken in bottom of slow cooker.
4. Add remaining ingredients.
5. Cook on low for 7 hours.

{preparation + cook time 7 hrs & 10 minutes **serves** 6**}**

Doug's Fireside Roast Chicken & Red Pepper Soup

4 cups roasted chicken breast, cubed
4 red bell peppers, seeded and diced
1 onion, peeled and diced
4 cloves garlic, peeled and minced
1 celery stalk, diced
1 cup tomato puree
3 cups low-sodium chicken broth
1 cup water
1/2 tsp nutmeg
1 tsp each sea salt and pepper
Extra virgin olive oil

1. Preheat oven to 400 degrees, coat roasting tray with olive oil.
2. Place bell pepper on tray and stick in oven for 20 minutes, turning halfway.
3. Place a dash of oil in a medium soup pot, sauté onions, celery and garlic.
4. Add roasted bell peppers and remaining ingredients to pot, bring to boil.
5. Reduce heat, simmer for 35 minutes.

{preparation + cook time 1 hr **serves** 4**}**

“Sniffles be gone” Orange Chicken Soup

1 lb chicken breast, bone-in, skinless, cubed
2 oranges, peeled segmented
1 lemon, juiced
2 carrots, peeled and sliced
1 onion, peeled and chopped
2 tbsp fresh ginger
2 cups low-sodium chicken stock
2 cups water
1 tsp rosemary
1 tsp each sea salt, white pepper
2 tbsp soy sauce
Extra virgin olive oil

1. Lightly coat 4 qt. slow cooker with extra virgin olive oil.
2. Place chicken in bottom of cooker, add remaining ingredients.
3. Cook on low for 8 hours.

{preparation + cook time 8 hrs **serves** 6**}**

Marg’s Chicken Tortilla Soup

2 chicken breasts, skinless, boneless, cubed
2 cups chopped tomatoes
1-1/2 cups corn
1 can black beans
1 jalapeno, seeded and sliced
1 onion, peeled and diced
4 cloves garlic, peeled and chopped
1 tsp oregano
1 tsp cumin
1 tsp each sea salt, black pepper
Extra virgin olive oil

Topping
Tortilla chips
½ cup sour cream

1. Heat olive oil in heavy pot. Add onions, garlic and sauté for a minute.
2. Add chicken and brown.
3. Add remaining ingredients save tortilla chips and cook on medium low for 30 minutes.
4. Top with a dollop of sour cream and crushed tortilla chips.

{preparation + cook time 1 hr **serves** 4**}**

Garlic Artichoke Chicken Soup

1/2 lb chicken breast, diced
2 cups sunchoke, chopped
1 red potato, peeled and chopped
1 carrot, peeled, sliced
1 green onion, sliced
2 cloves garlic, peeled and chopped
2 cups chicken stock
1/2 cup apple vinegar
1 tsp thyme
1 tsp each sea salt and coarse black pepper
Extra virgin olive oil

1. Heat Dutch oven to 375 degrees.
2. Add glug of oil, heat.
3. Add onions and garlic, sauté for one minute.
4. Add remaining ingredients, cover and cook for 45 minutes.

{preparation + cook time 1 hr **serves** 4**}**

Sue’s Luau Pineapple Chicken Soup

12 oz. chicken breast
1 tbsp ginger
1 red onion, diced
1 jalapeño, diced
1 tbsp lime juice
1/2 cup coriander leaves
3/4 cup pineapple
Extra virgin olive oil

1. Lightly coat 4 qt. slow cooker with olive oil.
2. Cube the chicken
3. Place chicken in bottom of slow cooker.
4. Add remaining ingredients in top.
5. Cook on low for 7 hours.

{preparation + cook time 7 1/2 hrs **serves** 4**}**

Grandma's Chicken Noodle Soup

1 lb chicken breast, skinless, bone-in, cubed
2 carrots, peeled and chopped
1 celery stalk, chopped
1 onion, peeled and chopped
4 cloves garlic, peeled and chopped
4 cups low-sodium chicken stock
1 cup fusilli noodles
1 tsp thyme
1 tsp each sea salt and pepper
Extra virgin olive oil

1. Heat olive oil in soup pot and brown chicken.
2. Add onions, garlic and veggies and cook until vegetables have slightly softened.
3. Pour in chicken stock and bring to boil, cover and simmer 20 minutes.
4. Add fusilli and cook for another 7 minutes.

{preparation + cook time 40 mins **serves** 4**}**

Saturday Caesar's Rice & Chicken Soup

1/2 lb chicken breast, skinless, boneless
1 green bell pepper, seeded and diced
2 medium tomatoes, chopped
1 onion, peeled and sliced
4 cloves garlic, peeled and chopped
1/2 cup rice
1 cup spicy V8 juice
¼ cup vodka
2 cups low-sodium chicken broth
1 tsp cayenne pepper
1 tsp each sea salt, black pepper
Extra virgin olive oil

1. Lightly coat 4 qt. slow cooker with olive oil.
2. Place chicken in bottom of cooker
3. Add remainder of ingredients.
4. Cook on medium high for 5 hours.

{preparation + cook time 5 ½ hrs **serves** 4**}**

Deconstructed Chicken Enchilada Soup

2 cups, roasted chicken, cubed
1 green bell pepper, seeded and diced
1 red bell pepper, seeded and diced
1 onion, peeled and diced
4 cloves garlic, peeled and diced
1 cup chicken stock
1 cup water
1 tsp Taco seasoning
1 tsp each, salt and pepper
Extra virgin olive oil

Cheese Sauce
3 tbsp butter
2 tbsp flour
2 cups cheddar cheese
1-1/2 cups milk

1. Heat a dash of olive oil in a medium-sized pot.
2. Add onion and garlic, cook until garlic is fragrant.
3. Add veggies, water and chicken stock, bring to boil.
4. Add cheese sauce (directions below) and remaining ingredients.
5. Cover and cook on medium-low for 10 minutes.

Cheese Sauce
In a saucepan melt butter, add flour and mix until it becomes a smooth paste.
Slowly pour in milk and blend in cheese until combined.

{preparation + cook time 1 hr **serves** 6**}**

Creamy Celery Root Chicken Soup

2 chicken breasts, boneless, skinless, cubed
1 celery root, peeled and grated
1 onion, peeled and chopped
1 tbsp fresh dill
2 tbsp butter
1/2 cup heavy cream
2 cups low-sodium chicken stock
1 tsp each sea salt, black pepper

1. Lightly coat 4 qt. slow cooker with olive oil.
2. Place chicken in bottom of slow cooker.
3. Add remaining ingredients.
4. Cook on low for 7 hours.

{preparation + cook time 7 ½ hrs **serves** 4**}**

Powerhouse Chicken Arugula Soup

½ lb chicken breasts, skinned and cubed
2 cups arugula, washed and chopped
1 russet potato, peeled and diced
2 onions, peeled and chopped
4 cloves garlic, peeled and chopped
2 cups chicken stock
1 cup water
½ tsp rosemary
1 tsp sea salt
1 tsp black pepper
2 tbsp butter

Topping
1 lemon, juiced

1. Melt butter in a heavy pot, add onion and cook until translucent.
2. Add chicken and sauté on high heat until brown
3. Add remaining ingredients, turn heat to medium low, cover and cook for 30 minutes.
4. Pour into bowls and squirt a little lemon on top.

{**preparation + cook time** 1 hr **serves** 4}

Parmesan Chicken Soup

1/2 lb chicken breast, boneless, skinless
1 onion, peeled and diced
4 cloves garlic, peeled and chopped
2 cups tomato puree
1 egg, whisked
1/4 cup parsley, chopped
1/2 cup parmesan, grated
1 tsp oregano
1 tsp each sea salt and black pepper

Topping
½ cup mozzarella, shredded

1. Lightly coat 4 qt. slow cooker with olive oil. Cube the chicken Place chicken in bottom of slow cooker. Add remaining ingredients.
2. Cook on medium for 4 hours.
3. Top with mozzarella and serve

{preparation + cook time 5 hrs **serves** 4**}**

Curried Chicken Soup

4 cups roasted chicken, cubed
1 medium onion, peeled and sliced
4 cloves garlic, peeled and minced
1 tbsp ginger, grated
1 cup tomato, pureed
1 tbsp tomato paste
2 cups chicken stock
1 cup water
1 tsp curry powder
1 tsp each salt and pepper
Extra virgin olive oil

Garnish
½ cup flat leaf parsley

1. Heat a dash of olive oil in medium pot, add onion and garlic and sauté until garlic is fragrant.
2. Add tomato paste, cook for one minute.
3. Add remaining ingredients, cover and cook on medium low for 25 minutes.
4. Top with parsley and serve

{preparation + cook time 40 mins **serves** 4-6**}**

Beef

Lumberjack Jack's Potato, Bacon, Olive Soup

1-1/2 lb potatoes
4 slices bacon, cooked and chopped into bits
1/2 cup Kalamata olives, pitted and sliced
1 onion, peeled and sliced
2 cups chicken broth
1/2 cup cream
1 cup milk
1 cup water
2 tbsp flour
1 tsp each sea salt, black pepper
Extra virgin olive oil

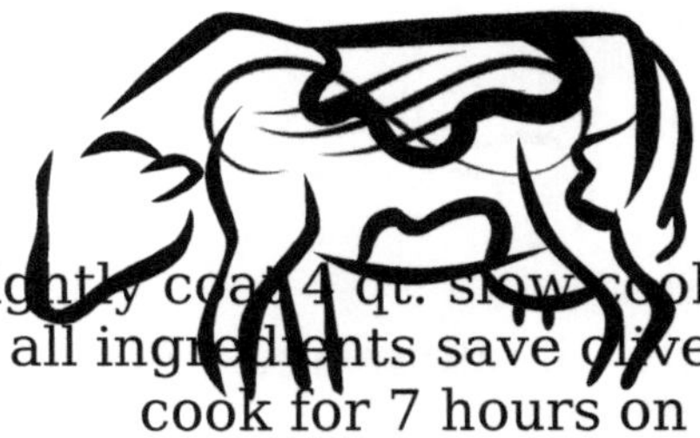

1. Lightly coat 4 qt. slow cooker with olive oil.
2. Place all ingredients save olives in slow cooker and cook for 7 hours on low.
3. Add olives, mix and serve.

{preparation + cook time 7 ½ hrs **serves** 4-6**}**

Deconstructed Cabbage Roll Soup

1 lb lean ground beef
1 medium cabbage, shredded
2 cups low-sodium chicken broth
2 cups tomatoes, pureed
1 onion, peeled and sliced
4 cloves garlic, peeled and chopped
1/2 cup rice
1 egg, beaten
1/4 cup milk
1/4 tsp cinnamon
2 tsp sugar
1 bay leaf
1 tsp each sea salt, black pepper
Extra virgin olive oil

1. Mix egg with sugar and 1/4 cup milk, set aside.
2. Heat olive oil in heavy pot, add onion and garlic, sauté for 2 minutes.
3. Add ground beef and brown.
4. Add remaining ingredients save egg mixture and bring to a boil.
5. Transfer to Dutch oven and slowly mix in egg mixture.
6. Cook in Dutch oven on medium for 1 hour at 350 degrees.

{preparation + cook time 1 ½ hrs **serves** 4**}**

Hearty Beef and Tomato Basil Soup

1/2 lb ground chuck
1 celery stalk, diced
2 carrots, peeled and sliced
3 cups pureed tomatoes
1 red onion, peeled and chopped
4 cloves garlic, minced
1/2 cup dry egg noodles
2 cups chicken stock
2 cups water
1/4 cup fresh basil, chopped
1/4 tsp cinnamon
1 tsp each sea salt, black pepper
Extra virgin olive oil

1. Heat 2 tbsp olive oil in heavy saucepan.
2. Add onions and sauté until translucent, add garlic and cook for a minute.
3. Add ground chuck and brown.
4. Stir in veggies and sauté until slightly softened
5. Add remaining ingredients, bring to boil.
6. Reduce heat, cover and allow to cook for 45 minutes.

{preparation + cook time 1 ½ hrs **serves** 4**}**

Beef Noodle Soup

½ lb beef steak, sliced against the grain
2 carrots, peeled and chopped
1/2 cup snap peas
2 cups egg noodles, dry
1 onion, peeled and chopped
4 cloves garlic, peeled and chopped
4 cups low-sodium beef stock
2 tbsp fresh basil, chopped
1 tsp cinnamon
1 tsp cayenne pepper
1 tsp each sea salt and pepper
Extra virgin olive oil

1. Heat olive oil in soup pot and brown beef, set aside
2. Add onions, garlic and veggies and cook until vegetables have slightly softened.
3. Pour in beef stock and bring to boil, cover and simmer 20 minutes.
4. Add egg noodles, beef and basil and cook for another 7 minutes.

{preparation + cook time 1 hr **serves** 4**}**

Mexican Party Soup

1/2 lb lean ground beef
1 cup corn kernels
1 jalapeno, seeded and minced
1 green bell pepper, seeded and diced
2 cups tomatoes, diced
2 cups beef stock
1/2 cup cheddar, shredded
¼ cup olives, pitted and sliced
1 onion, peeled and diced
4 cloves garlic, peeled and minced
1 tsp each, salt and pepper
Extra virgin olive oil

1. Heat 3 tbsp olive oil in heavy pot.
2. Sauté onions and garlic for a minute.
3. Add beef, sauté until browned.
4. Add remaining ingredients save cheddar cheese and olives.
5. Cover and cook for 30 minutes on medium low.
6. Top with cheddar cheese and olives.

{preparation + cook time 1 hr **serves** 4-6**}**

Thai Beef Soup

1 lb top round, cubed
1 red bell pepper, seeded and diced
2 medium tomatoes, chopped
2 cups low-sodium chicken broth
½ cup coconut milk
1 onion, peeled and sliced
1 tbsp ginger, grated
1/2 cup rice
1 tsp curry powder
1 tsp cayenne pepper
1 tsp each sea salt, black pepper
Extra virgin olive oil

1. Lightly coat 4 qt. slow cooker with olive oil.
2. Place beef in bottom of cooker
3. Add remainder of ingredients.
4. Cook on low for 8 hours.

{preparation + cook time 9 hrs **serves** 6**}**

Spur-Kickin' Chili

1 lbs ground chuck
1-1/2 lb sirloin, cubed
1 jalapeno, peeled and sliced
1 green chilli pepper, minced
2 cups tomato puree
2 onions, peeled and sliced
6 cloves garlic, peeled and minced
¼ cup tequila
2 tbsp brown sugar
2 cups beef stock
2 cups water
1 tbsp cumin
1 tbsp oregano
1 tsp each sea salt, black pepper
Extra virgin olive oil

1. Heat a dash of olive oil in large soup pot.
2. Add onions and garlic until garlic is fragrant.
3. Add sirloin and brown, set aside.
4. Add ground chuck, brown.
5. Stir in onion, garlic, peppers and cook for two minutes.
6. Add remaining ingredients, turn heat to medium low, cover and cook for 45 minutes.

{preparation + cook time 1 ½ hrs **serves** 6**}**

The Ranch Hand's Steak Indulgence

1/2 lb sirloin steak, thinly sliced
1 cup fingerling potatoes, peeled
1 cup baby carrots
2 cloves garlic, peeled and chopped
1 red onion, peeled and chopped.
1/2 cup red wine
2 cups low-sodium chicken broth
1 tsp rosemary
1 tsp cracked black pepper
Extra virgin olive oil

1. Heat a dash of olive oil in a soup pot over medium heat.
2. Cook steak 30 seconds per side.
3. Add garlic and onion, cook for one minute.
4. Mix in carrots and potatoes.
5. Add remaining ingredients and cook on medium low for one hour.

{preparation + cook time 2 hrs **serves** 6**}**

Brock's Beef and Broccoli Soup

1/2 lb top round
4 cups broccoli florets
1/2 cup bulgur
1 onion, peeled and chopped
1 tsp rosemary
2 cups low-sodium chicken stock
1 tsp each sea salt, black pepper

1. Lightly coat 4 qt. slow cooker with olive oil.
2. Place beef in bottom of slow cooker.
3. Add remaining ingredients.
4. Cook on low for 7 hours.

{preparation + cook time 7 ½ hrs **serves** 6**}**

Philly Cheesesteak in a Bowl

1/2 lb strip loin, thinly sliced
1 cup portabella mushrooms, sliced
1 green bell pepper, seeded and diced
4 cloves garlic, peeled and chopped
1 onion, peeled and diced
2 cups low-sodium beef stock
1 cup water
¾ cup provolone cheese, grated
1 tsp each sea salt and black pepper
1 tbsp butter
1 tbsp flour
1 cup milk, heated
Extra virgin olive oil

1. Melt butter in a saucepan, add butter and mix until you have a paste.
2. Slowly whisk in milk.
3. Remove from heat and mix in cheese until well combined.
4. Place a dash of extra virgin olive oil in Dutch Oven at 350 degrees.
5. Sauté strip loin for 30 seconds per side.
6. Add onion, garlic and veggies, sauté for three minutes.
7. Add remaining ingredients include provolone sauce and cook on 300 for one hour.

{preparation + cook time 2 hrs **serves** 4**}**

Beef and Chickpea Yogurt Soup

1/2 lb top round, thinly sliced
2 cups chickpeas, prepared
1 medium onion, peeled and chopped
4 cloves garlic, peeled and chopped
1/2 cup tomato puree
1 cup Greek yogurt
1 egg
1 tsp cayenne pepper
1 tsp oregano
1 tsp each sea salt, black pepper
Extra virgin olive oil

1. Mix egg and yogurt, set aside
2. Heat olive oil in heavy pan, add beef and cook 30 seconds per side.
3. Remove beef, set aside.
4. Add onions and garlic, sauté for one minute.
5. Stir in chickpeas and chicken stock.
6. Slowly add egg mixture followed by remaining ingredients including beef.

Cover and cook for one hour on medium low

{preparation + cook time 1 1/2 hrs **serves** 4**}**

The Italian Bride's Parmesan Chicken Soup

1/2 lb chicken breast, boneless, skinless, cubed
1 onion, peeled and diced
4 cloves garlic, peeled and chopped
2 cups tomato puree
1 egg, whisked
1/4 cup parsley, chopped
1/2 cup parmesan, grated
1 tsp oregano
1 tsp each sea salt and black pepper

Topping
½ cup mozzarella, shredded

1. Lightly coat 4 qt. slow cooker with olive oil.
2. Place chicken in bottom of slow cooker.
3. Add remaining ingredients.
4. Cook on medium for 4 hours.
5. Top with mozzarella and serve

{preparation + cook time 4 1/2 hrs **serves** 4**}**

Turkey

Thanksgiving in July Soup

1 lb ground turkey
2 celery stalks, diced
2 carrots, peeled and sliced
1 potato, peeled and chopped
½ cup dried cranberries
1 red onion, peeled and chopped
4 cloves garlic, minced
3 cups pureed tomatoes
6 cups chicken stock
2 cups water
1 tsp each sea salt, black pepper
Extra virgin olive oil

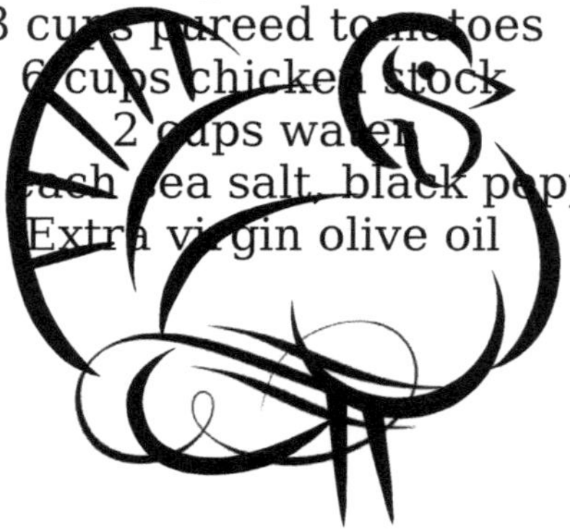

1. Heat 2 tbsp olive oil in heavy saucepan.
2. Add onions and sauté until translucent, add garlic and cook for a minute.
3. Add turkey and brown.
4. Stir in remaining veggies and sauté for five minutes.
5. Add remaining ingredients, cover and allow to cook for 45 minutes.

{preparation + cook time 1 1/2 hrs **serves** 6-8**}**

Hearty White Bean and Turkey Soup

½ lb turkey breast, skinless, boneless
2 red potatoes, peeled and cut in 1/8
1 celery stalk, sliced
½ cup white beans
1 onion, peeled and sliced
4 cloves garlic, peeled and chopped
2 cups low-sodium chicken broth
1 cup tomatoes, pureed.
1 cup water
1 tsp cayenne pepper
1 bay leaf
1 tsp each sea salt, black pepper
Extra virgin olive oil

1. Lightly coat slow cooker with olive oil.
2. Place turkey breast in bottom of cooker,
3. Add remainder of ingredients.
4. Cook on low for 7 hours.
5. Remove bay leaf before serving.

{preparation + cook time 7 1/2 hrs **serves** 4-6**}**

The Turkey Club Soup

1 turkey breast, boneless, skinless, sliced
6 slices turkey bacon, cooked and chopped
1 red onion, peeled and chopped.
1 tomato, chopped
1 cup tomato, pureed
2 cups low-sodium chicken broth
Extra virgin olive oil

1. Lightly coat 4 qt. slow cooker with olive oil.
2. Place turkey in bottom of slow cooker.
3. Add remaining ingredients.
4. Cook on low for 7 hours.

{preparation + cook time 7 1/2 hrs **serves** 6**}**

Harvest Pumpkin and Turkey Soup

3 cups, turkey, cooked and diced
1 cup pumpkin, diced
1 onion, peeled and chopped
4 cloves garlic, peeled and chopped
2 tbsp butter
2 cups low-sodium chicken or turkey stock
1 tsp each sea salt, black pepper

1. Lightly coat 4 qt. slow cooker with olive oil.
2. Mix all items together in slow cooker.
3. Cook on medium-low for 5 hours.

{preparation + cook time 5 1/2 hrs **serves** 4**}**

Gramps' Split Pea and Turkey Soup

1-½ cups roast turkey, cubed
1 cup split peas
1-½ cups tomato puree
1 red onion, peeled and chopped
2 cups low-sodium beef broth
1 tsp balsamic vinegar
1 tsp rosemary
1 tsp each sea salt and pepper

1. Lightly coat 4 qt. slow cooker with olive oil.
2. Place ingredients in slow cooker and cook on low for 7 hours.

{preparation + cook time 7 1/2 hrs **serves** 4**}**

Pork

Lily's Special Leek and Sausage Soup

2 cups leek, chopped
1/2 lb turkey sausage, casings removed
1 russet potato, peeled and diced
1 pear, peeled, cored and cubed
2 slices bacon, cooked and chopped into bits
1 onion, peeled and sliced
2 cups chicken broth
1 cup water
1 tsp each sea salt, black pepper
Extra virgin olive oil

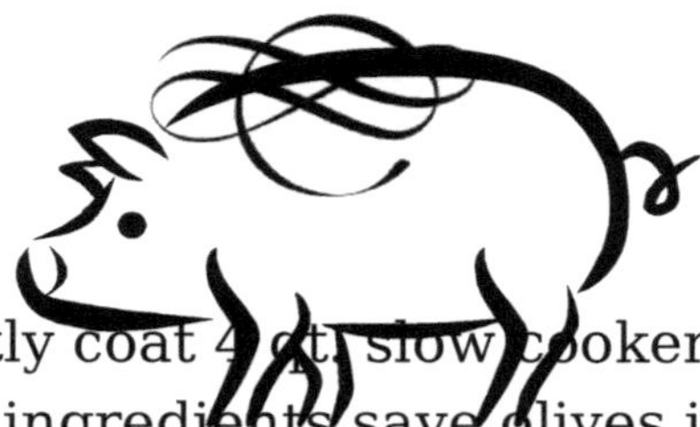

1. Lightly coat 4 qt. slow cooker with olive oil.
2. Place all ingredients save olives in slow cooker and cook for 7 hours on low.
3. Add olives, mix and serve.

{preparation + cook time 7 1/2 hrs **serves** 4-6**}**

Turnip Meets Bacon

6 medium turnips, peeled and diced
4 slices cooked bacon, chopped
1 onion, peeled and diced
1/2 cup cream
2 cups low-sodium chicken broth
1 cup water
1/2 tsp rosemary
1 tsp each sea salt, black pepper

1. Place all ingredients in cooker.
2. Turn to low and cook for 7 hours.

{preparation + cook time 7 1/2 hrs **serves** 4**}**

Pork, Apple and Cabbage Goodness Soup

1 lb lean ground pork
4 cups cabbage, shredded
1 apple, peeled, cored, cubed
2 cups low-sodium chicken broth
1 potato, peeled and diced
1 onion, peeled and sliced
1 tsp rosemary
1 tsp sugar
1 bay leaf
1 tsp each sea salt, black pepper
Extra virgin olive oil

1. Heat olive oil in heavy pot, add onion and garlic, sauté for 2 minutes.
2. Add ground pork and brown.
3. Add remaining ingredients and bring to a boil.
4. Transfer to Dutch oven and cook on medium for 1 hour at 350 degrees.

{preparation + cook time 1 1/2 hrs **serves** 4**}**

Maple-Roasted Ham and Cheese Soup

2 cups, maple-roasted ham, cubed
1 russet potato, peeled and diced
1 carrot, peeled and sliced
1 celery stalk, diced
1 green onion, diced
2 tbsp butter
1 tbsp flour
1-1/2 cups cheddar cheese
1-1/2 cups milk
1 cup chicken stock
1 cup water
1 tsp each, salt and pepper
Extra virgin olive oil

1. Heat a dash of olive oil in a medium-sized pot.
2. Add onion and cook until translucent.
3. Add veggies, water and chicken stock, bring to boil.
4. In a saucepan melt butter, add flour and mix until it becomes a smooth paste.
5. Slowly pour in milk and bring to a boil.
6. Add cheese and remaining ingredients and mix until cheese is melted.
7. Add cheese sauce and ham to veggies.
8. Cover and cook on medium-low for 7 minutes.

{preparation + cook time 1 hr **serves** 6**}**

Cheesy Bacon and Pea Soup

8 slices bacon, cooked and sliced
1 cup peas
1 russet potato, peeled and diced
1 carrot, peeled and sliced
1 celery stalk, diced
1 green onion, diced
1 cup beef stock
1 cup water
1 tsp each, salt and pepper
Extra virgin olive oil

Cheese Sauce
2 tbsp butter
1 tbsp flour
1-1/2 cups cheddar cheese
1-1/2 cups milk

1. Heat 2 tbsp olive oil in a heavy pot.

2. Add onion and cook until translucent.

3. Add veggies, water and beef stock, bring to boil.

4. In a saucepan melt butter, add flour and mix until it becomes a smooth paste.

5. Slowly pour in milk and bring to a boil.

6. Add cheese and remaining ingredients and mix until cheese is melted.

7. Add cheese sauce and bacon to veggies.

8. Cover and cook on medium-low for 7 minutes.

{preparation + cook time 1 hr **serves** 6**}**

Spicy Sausage and Gnocchi Soup

1/2 lb spicy pork sausage, casings removed
1 red onion, peeled and chopped
4 cloves garlic, peeled and minced
1/2 lb parmesan gnocchi
1 cup tomatoes, pureed
2 cups vegetable stock
1/4 cup parmesan
Extra virgin olive oil

1. Heat a dash of olive oil in a heavy pot over medium heat.
2. Sauté pork sausage until browned, add onions and garlic and sauté until garlic is fragrant.
3. Add remaining ingredients save parmesan and bring to boil.
4. Simmer for 10 minutes, sprinkle with cheese.

{preparation + cook time 40mins **serves** 4**}**

Wonton Soup

Wrappers
1/2 lb pork loin, chopped
4 cloves garlic peeled and minced
1 green onion, minced
1 tbsp low sodium soy sauce
1 tbsp fish sauce
1 tsp brown sugar
18 wonton wrappers

Soup
4 cups chicken stock

1. Mix together all ingredients save wonton wrappers.
2. Drop a small amount of the pork mixture in each wrapper and fold to make a triangle, moisten with water and press down with fingers to seal.
3. Pour chicken stock into heavy medium-sized pan and bring to boil.
4. Place wontons in chicken stock and allow to cook for 7 minutes.

{preparation + cook time 40mins **serves** 6**}**

Poland says Hello Soup

1/2 lb Polish Kielbasa
1 red bell pepper, seeded and diced
1/2 medium cabbage, shredded
2 cloves garlic, peeled and diced
2 cups chicken stock
2 cups water
1 tsp each sea salt, ground black pepper
Extra virgin olive oil

1. Heat 1 tbsp oil in soup pot.
2. Add onions and kielbasa, sauté for 3 minutes.
3. Add garlic, sauté one minute.
4. Reduce heat to low, add remaining ingredients.
5. Cook for 30 minutes

{preparation + cook time 40mins **serves** 4**}**

Hoity-Toity Bacon French Onion Soup

4 slices bacon, cooked and chopped
1 white onions, chopped and diced
2 sweet onions, chopped and diced
1/2 cup white wine, dry
4 cups low-sodium beef broth
2 cups water
1 tsp thyme
1 tsp each salt, white pepper
1 cup Swiss cheese, grated
2 cups French bread, cubed
Extra virgin olive oil

1. Heat olive oil in heavy pan on medium and add onions, sauté until translucent.
2. Add wine, beef broth and thyme, bring to boil.
3. Reduce heat to low and cook for 30 minutes.
4. While waiting toast bread cubes in a tbsp of butter in saucepan.
5. Preheat broiler
6. Place 6 soup bowls on cookie sheet and add toasted bread cubes per cup.
7. Top with soup mixture and sprinkle with cheese.
8. Place in broiler for 7 minutes.

{preparation + cook time 1 hr **serves** 6**}**

Ground Pork and Bean Soup

½ lb ground pork
2 cups white beans
2 green onions, sliced
4 cloves garlic, peeled and minced
1 cup tomato, pureed
2 cups chicken stock
1 cup water
1 tsp oregano
1 tsp cayenne
1 tsp each salt and pepper
Extra virgin olive oil

1. Heat a dash of olive oil in medium pot, add cumin, green onion and garlic and sauté until garlic is fragrant.
2. Add ground pork and sauté until browned.
3. Lightly coat a 4 oz slow cooker with olive oil.
4. Place all ingredients including cooked pork mixture in slow cooker.
5. Cook on medium low for 5 hours.

{preparation + cook time 5 ½ hrs **serves** 4-6**}**

Vegetable

Cottontail's Roasted Carrot Soup

1 lb carrots, peeled and diced
1 sweet onion, peeled and diced
1 tbsp ginger, grated
1 celery stalk, diced
1 medium potato, peeled and diced
3 cups low-sodium chicken broth
1 cup water
1/2 tsp nutmeg
1 tsp each sea salt and pepper
Extra virgin olive oil

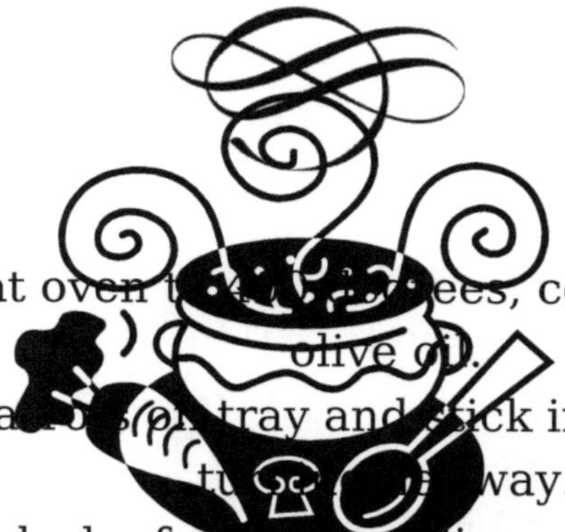

1. Preheat oven to 400 degrees, coat roasting tray with olive oil.

2. Place carrots on tray and stick in oven for 30 minutes, turning halfway.

3. Place a dash of oil in a medium soup pot, sauté onions, celery and ginger.

4. Add roast carrots and remaining ingredients to pot, bring to boil.

5. Reduce heat, simmer for 35 minutes.

6. Using hand immersion blender, blend.

{preparation + cook time 1 ½ hrs **serves** 4**}**

Bessie's Favourite Green Bean Soup

1 lb green beans, trimmed and chopped
4 cloves garlic, peeled and minced
2 tbsp butter
2 tbsp flour
1 tsp paprika
2 cups low-fat chicken stock
1 cup low-fat sour cream
1 tsp each sea salt, black pepper

1. In soup pot, melt 1 tbsp butter and sauté garlic until fragrant.
2. Add green beans and sauté for five minutes.
3. Add chicken broth and bring to boil. Reduce heat and simmer for 20 minutes.
4. In saucepan, melt 2 tbsp butter and mix in flour until it forms paste and whisk in sour cream.
5. Ladle some hot liquid from green beans into sour cream mixture.
6. Slowly add sour cream mixture to green beans.
7. Cover and simmer on low.

{preparation + cook time 1 ½ hrs **serves** 4**}**

Roast Garlic and Mushroom Soup

1 lb wild mushrooms
3 large bulbs garlic
2 red onions, peeled and chopped
1/4 cup fresh basil, chopped
2 cups French bread, cubed
1 lemon, juiced
1 cup heavy cream
3 cups low-sodium chicken stock
1 tsp oregano
1 tsp each sea salt and black pepper
Extra virgin olive oil

1. Preheat oven at 375 degrees and lightly coat roasting tray with olive oil.
2. Place garlic bulbs, skin on, on tray, drizzle with olive oil and roast for 10 minutes.
3. Remove skins from roasted garlic and mix up roasted garlic into paste.
4. Heat Dutch oven to 375 degrees.
5. Add glug of olive oil and sauté onions and mushrooms.
6. Mix in remaining ingredients including garlic paste.
7. Cover and cook for 45 minutes.

{**preparation + cook time** 1 ½ hrs **serves** 6-8}

Sweet Potato and Blue Cheese Soup

2 large sweet potatoes, peeled and cubed
1/2 cup blue cheese, crumbled
1 onion, peeled and sliced
2 cups chicken broth
1/2 cup cream
1 cup milk
1 cup water
2 tbsp flour
1 tsp each sea salt, black pepper
Extra virgin olive oil

1. Lightly coat 4 qt. slow cooker with olive oil.
2. Place all ingredients in slow cooker and cook for 8 hours on low.

{preparation + cook time 8 ½ hrs **serves** 4-6**}**

French Onion Deliciousness

2 white onions, chopped and diced
2 sweet onions, chopped and diced
1/2 cup white wine, dry
6 cups low-sodium beef broth
2 cups water
1 tsp thyme
1 tsp each salt, white pepper
1 cup Swiss cheese, grated
2 cups French bread, cubed
Extra virgin olive oil

1. Heat olive oil in heavy pan on medium and add onions, sauté until translucent.
2. Add wine, beef broth and thyme, bring to boil.
3. Reduce heat to low and cook for 30 minutes.
4. Lightly coat baking sheet with oil and toast bread in oven at 375 degrees until golden.
5. Preheat broiler
6. Place 6 soup bowls on cookie sheet and add toasted bread cubes per cup.
7. Top with soup mixture and sprinkle with cheese.
8. Place in broiler for 7 minutes.

{preparation + cook time 1 ½ hrs **serves** 6**}**

Easy Red Lentil Soup

2 cups red lentils
1 red onion, peeled and sliced
3 cloves garlic, peeled and minced
1/2 tsp oregano
1 tbsp tomato paste
3 cups low-sodium chicken stock
1 tsp each salt and pepper
1 lemon, juiced
Extra virgin olive oil

1. Wash lentils and allow them to sit on hot water for 1/2 an hour.
2. Heat a dash of olive oil in medium pot, add onion and garlic and sauté until garlic is fragrant.
3. Add tomato paste, cook for one minute.
4. Add remaining ingredients, cover and cook on medium low for 25 minutes.
5. Using a hand immersion blender, mix until smooth.

{preparation + cook time 1 ½ hrs **serves** 4**}**

Curried Chickpea Soup

4 cups chickpeas, prepared
1 medium onion, peeled and sliced
5 cloves garlic, peeled and minced
1 tbsp ginger, grated
1 tsp curry powder
1 cup tomato, pureed
1 tbsp tomato paste
2 cups vegetable stock
1 cup water
1 tsp each salt and pepper
Extra virgin olive oil

1. Wash chickpeas.
2. Heat a dash of olive oil in medium pot, add onion and garlic and sauté until garlic is fragrant.
3. Add tomato paste, cook for one minute.
4. Add remaining ingredients, cover and cook on medium low for 25 minutes.
5. Using a hand immersion blender, mix until smooth.

{preparation + cook time 1 ½ hrs **serves** 4-6**}**

White bean and Carrot Soup

4 cups white beans
2 carrots, peeled and sliced
2 green onions, sliced
5 cloves garlic, peeled and minced
1 cup tomato, pureed
1 tbsp tomato paste
2 cups vegetable stock
1 cup water
1 tsp cumin
1 tsp oregano
1 tsp cayenne
1 tsp each salt and pepper
Extra virgin olive oil

1. Heat a dash of olive oil in medium pot, add cumin, green onion and garlic and sauté until garlic is fragrant.
2. Lightly coat a 4 oz slow cooker with olive oil.
3. Place all ingredients including cooked onion mixture in slow cooker.
4. Cook on medium low for 5 hours.

{preparation + cook time 5 ½ hrs **serves** 4-6**}**

Broccoli and Kale Soup

2 lbs broccoli, chopped
2 cups kale, washed and chopped
1 onion, peeled and diced
2 tbsp flour
2 cups low-sodium chicken broth
2 cups water
1/2 cup cream
1 tsp each sea salt, cracked black pepper

1. Melt butter in medium soup pot.
2. Add onion and sauté until translucent.
3. Add, kale and broccoli and sauté until you can smell the broccoli.
4. Sprinkle in flour and cook for two minutes.
5. Stir in remaining ingredients and cook on low for 30 minutes.
6. Cool, pour into blender and mix until smooth.

{preparation + cook time 1 hr **serves** 4**}**

Potato and Cheese Comfort

2 lbs potatoes peeled and diced
2 cups shredded jack cheese
1 carrot, peeled and shredded
1 onion, peeled and diced
2 tbsp flour
2 cups low-sodium chicken broth
2 cups water
1/2 cup cream
1 tsp each sea salt, cracked black pepper

1. Melt butter in medium soup pot.
2. Add onion and sauté until translucent.
3. Add flour and cook for a minute.
4. Stir in remaining ingredients and cook on low for 30 minutes.
5. Using an immersion blender, mix until smooth.

{preparation + cook time 1 hr **serves** 6**}**

Autumn Harvest Squash Soup

1 butternut squash, halved and seeded
2 red bell peppers, halved and seeded
1 onion, peeled and diced
4 cloves garlic, peeled and minced
1/2 cup cream
1 tsp each sea salt, black pepper
Extra virgin olive oil

1. Preheat oven to 425 degrees and lightly coat with olive oil.
2. Wrap two halves of squash together in aluminium foil.
3. Place squash and bell pepper on baking tray and roast for 30 minutes.
4. Cool, remove skin from squash and dice. Slice bell pepper.
5. Heat 2 tbsp olive oil in medium soup pot, add onion and sauté until translucent.
6. Add remaining ingredients, cover and cook for 45 minutes.

{preparation + cook time 1 1/2 hrs **serves** 4**}**

Creamy Pea Soup

2 cups green peas
1 onion, peeled and chopped
4 cloves garlic, peeled and chopped
2 potatoes,peeled and chopped
3 cups vegetable stock
1/2 cup heavy cream
2 tbsp butter
1 tsp each sea salt, black pepper

1. Heat butter in a saucepan and sauté onions and garlic until the garlic is fragrant.
2. Place onion and garlic in a 4 qt. slow cooker, add remaining ingredients and cook on low for 8 7 hours.
3. Using a hand immersion blender, blend smooth until smooth.

{preparation + cook time 7 1/2 hrs **serves** 4**}**

Sleigh Ride Mushroom Soup

4 cups Portobello mushrooms
1/4 cup porcini mushrooms, chopped
1 red onion, peeled and sliced
4 cloves garlic, peeled and chopped
3 cups low-sodium chicken stock
½ cup heavy cream
3 tbsp flour
1 tsp thyme
1/2 tsp nutmeg
1 tsp sea salt
Extra virgin olive oil

1. Dilute flour with some water.
2. Heat 3 tbsp extra virgin olive oil in a heavy pot.
3. Add onions, garlic and sauté for two minutes.
4. Add mushrooms and sauté until moisture is released.
5. Add chicken broth and bring to a boil, simmer 10 minutes.
6. Slowly stir in flour mixture.
7. Add remaining ingredients, cover and simmer on low for 20 minutes.

{preparation + cook time 1 1/2 hrs **serves** 4**}**

Brilliant Tomato and Sweet Potato Soup

2 cups diced tomatoes
1 onion, peeled and chopped
4 cloves garlic, peeled and chopped
2 sweet potatoes,peeled and chopped
3 cups chicken stock
1/2 cup heavy cream
2 tbsp butter
1 bay leaf
1 tsp oregano
1 tsp each sea salt, black pepper

1. Heat butter in a saucepan and sauté onions and garlic until the garlic is fragrant.

2. Place onion and garlic in a 4 qt. slow cooker, add remaining ingredients and cook on low for 8 7 hours.

3. Remove bay leaf.

4. Using a hand immersion blender, blend smooth until smooth.

{preparation + cook time 7 1/2 hrs **serves** 4**}**

Asparagus Potato Soup

2 medium potatoes, peeled and chopped
1 bunch asparagus, washed and trimmed
1 onion, peeled and chopped
3 cloves garlic, peeled and chopped
3 cups low-sodium chicken stock
1 lemon, juiced
2 tbsp butter
1 tsp rosemary
1 tsp each sea salt, white pepper
Extra virgin olive oil

1. Lightly coat 4 qt. slow cooker with extra virgin olive oil.
2. Chop asparagus into bite-size pieces.
3. Place all ingredients in slow cooker and cook on low for 8 hours.

{preparation + cook time 8 1/2 hrs **serves** 4**}**

Railroad Rice and Beans

1-½ cups red kidney beans
1 cup long-grained rice
1-½ cups tomato, diced
1 red onion, peeled and chopped
3 cloves garlic, peeled and chopped
2 cups low-sodium beef broth
1 tsp oregano
½ tsp cumin
1 tsp each sea salt and pepper.

1. Lightly coat 4 qt. slow cooker with olive oil.
2. Place ingredients in slow cooker and cook on low for 7 hours

{preparation + cook time 7 1/2 hrs **serves** 2**}**

Healthy Rice and Lentil Soup

2 cups black lentils
2 green onions, sliced
4 cloves garlic, peeled and minced
1 tsp ginger, ground
½ cup rice
2 tbsp tomato paste
2 cups chicken stock
1 cup water
1 tsp cumin
1 tsp coriander
1 tsp each salt and pepper
Extra virgin olive oil

1. Heat a dash of olive oil in medium pot, add cumin, green onion and garlic and sauté until garlic is fragrant.

2. Add tomato paste and cook for two minutes.

3. Add remaining ingredients.

4. Cover and cook on medium low for 25 minutes.

{preparation + cook time 45 mins **serves** 4-6**}**

Zucchini and Dill White Bean Soup

1 cup zucchini, chopped
2 cups white beans
1 red onion, peeled and sliced
4 cloves garlic, peeled and minced
2 tsp fresh dill
1 cup tomato, pureed
1 tbsp tomato paste
2 cups vegetable stock
1 tsp cayenne
1 tsp each salt and pepper
Extra virgin olive oil

1. Heat a dash of olive oil in medium pot, add onion and garlic and sauté until garlic is fragrant.
2. Lightly coat a 4 oz slow cooker with olive oil.
3. Place all ingredients including cooked onion mixture in slow cooker.
4. Cook on medium low for 5 hours.

{preparation + cook time 5 1/2 hrs **serves** 4-6**}**

Colours of Fall Squash Soup

1 acorn squash, peeled, seeded and chopped
2 red bell peppers
1 onion, diced
2 tbsp grated ginger
2 cups low-sodium chicken broth
½ cup heavy cream
1 tsp cayenne pepper
1 tsp each sea salt, coarse black pepper
Extra virgin olive oil

1. Lightly coat 4 qt. slow cooker with olive oil.
2. Mix ingredients together in slow cooker.
3. Cook on low for 7 hours.
4. Cool until safe to handle.
5. Pour into blender and mix until smooth.

{preparation + cook time 7 1/2 hrs **serves** 6**}**

Decadent Asiago Cauliflower Soup

1 medium cauliflower, sliced into florets
1 carrot, peeled and sliced
1 red onion, peeled and sliced
1/2 cup Asiago cheese
1 cup sour cream
2 cups chicken broth
1 cup water
1 tsp sea salt
1 tsp white pepper
Extra virgin olive oil

1. Lightly coat 4 qt. slow cooker with olive oil.
2. Combine ingredients in slow cooker.
3. Cook on medium low for 5 hours.
4. Using hand immersion blender, mix until smooth.

{preparation + cook time 5 1/2 hrs **serves** 4**}**

Cauliflower and Blue Cheese Soup

1 medium cauliflower, separated into florets
1/2 cup blue cheese, crumbled
1 onion, peeled and sliced
2 cups chicken broth
1/2 cup cream
1 cup milk
1 cup water
2 tbsp butter
2 tbsp flour
1 tsp each sea salt, black pepper
Extra virgin olive oil

1. In a medium saucepan melt butter, mix in butter until it forms paste.
2. Add milk and cheese, mix until smooth.
3. Place a dash of oil in a soup pot and sauté onions, garlic.
4. Add remaining ingredients including cheese mixture and cook on low for one hour.
5. Using hand immersion blender, mix until smooth.

{preparation + cook time 1 hr **serves** 4-6**}**

Parmesan Zucchini Soup

4 cups zucchini, sliced
1 carrot, peeled and sliced
1 green onion, peeled and sliced
1/2 cup parmesan
1 cup sour cream
3 cups chicken broth
1 tsp oregano
1 tsp sea salt
1 tsp white pepper
Extra virgin olive oil

1. Lightly coat 4 qt. slow cooker with olive oil.
2. Combine ingredients in slow cooker.
3. Cook on medium low for 5 hours.

{preparation + cook time 5 1/2 hrs **serves** 4**}**

Carolina's Corn Chowder

1 lb corn kernels
1 green onion, chopped
1 carrot, peeled and sliced
1 celery, sliced
1 red bell pepper, seeded and diced
1 russet potato, peeled and sliced
1/2 cup heavy cream
1/4 cup flat leaf parsley, chopped
2 cups chicken broth

1. Combine all items save cream in 4 qt. slow cooker.
2. Cook on low for 7 hours on low.
3. Stir in cream and cook for 10 minutes.

{preparation + cook time 7 1/2 hrs **serves** 4**}**

Lime Zinger Soup

2 tomatoes, chopped
1 celery stalk, diced
1 onion, peeled and chopped
1 can tomato paste
1 lime, juiced
1 cup V8 juice
2 cups low-sodium chicken stock

1. Combine ingredients in 4 qt. slow cooker.
2. Cook on low for 8 hours
3. 1 tsp sea salt and pepper

{preparation + cook time 8 1/2 hrs **serves** 4**}**

Mushroom Medley Soup

2 cups Portobella mushrooms
1 cup chanterelles
1/4 cup porcini mushrooms
1 red onion, peeled and sliced
4 cloves garlic, peeled and chopped
1/4 cup parsley leaves, chopped
3 cups vegetable stock
1 tsp thyme
1/2 tsp nutmeg
1 tsp sea salt
Extra virgin olive oil

1. Chop up porcini mushrooms, place in small dish and cover with hot water, set aside.
2. Heat 3 tbsp extra virgin olive oil in a heavy pot.
3. Add onions, garlic and sauté for two minutes.
4. Add mushrooms and sauté for another five minutes.
5. Add remaining ingredients, cover and cook for 30 minutes.
6. Using a hand immersion blender, blend soup for just over a minute so soup remains chunky with a slightly thick base

{preparation + cook time 1 1/2 hrs **serves** 4**}**

Broths

Delicious Chicken Broth

7 lbs roasting chickens
2 onions, peeled and sliced
10 cloves garlic, peeled
3 carrots, peeled and sliced
2 celery stalks peeled and sliced
1/4 cup flat-leaf parsley
1/4 cup thyme
1/4 cup dill

1. Place ingredients in 4 qt. slow cooker and cover with water.
2. [illegible] h for one hour.
3. Reduce heat and cook on low for 10 hours.
4. Strain [illegible] layer, refrigerate if using [illegible] or freeze.

{preparation + cook time 10 1/2 hrs **makes** 4 cups**}**

Easy Chicken Broth

1 chicken carcass
1 onion, peeled and rough-chopped
1 carrot, peeled and chopped
1 celery stalk, chopped
5 black peppercorns
6 cups water

1. Place bones and water in large stock pot, bring to boil.
2. Reduce heat and simmer for 45 minutes.
3. Remove fat layer on top of bone stock.
4. Add vegetables
5. Allow vegetables and carcass to combine flavours for 30 minutes.
6. Strain and compost veggies.

{preparation + cook time 2 hrs **makes** 2 cups**}**

Absolute Basic Beef Broth

1 lb beef bones
1 onion, peeled and chopped
1 celery stalk, chopped
1 carrot, peeled and chopped
1 parsnip, peeled and chopped
Water

1. Place bones, veggies and enough water to cover everything twice over in a large stock pot.
2. Bring to boil.
3. Reduce heat and simmer for 12 hours.
4. Strain.

{**preparation + cook time** 12 ½ hrs **makes** 4 cups}

Scotch Broth

1 lb beef bones with meat
1 carrot, peeled and sliced
1 celery stalk, chopped
1 onion, peeled and chopped
3 tbsp barley
8 cups water
1 bay leaf
Extra virgin olive oil

1. Lightly coat slow cooker with olive oil.
2. Mix together ingredients in soup pot.
3. Cook on medium low for 6 hours.
4. Strain.

{preparation + cook time 6 ½ hrs **makes** 4 cups**}**

Delicious Vegetable Broth

1/2 lb celery, diced
1/2 lb carrots, peeled, diced
4 green bell peppers, seeded and chopped
4 red bell peppers, seeded and chopped
4 tomatoes, chopped
2 onions, peeled and sliced
6 cloves garlic, peeled and chopped
10 peppercorns
1 bay leaf
Water
Extra virgin olive oil

1. Preheat oven to 400 degrees and coat roasting pan with olive oil.
2. Place veggies in roasting pan and cook for 10 minutes.
3. Cover with aluminium foil and cook for another 30 minutes.
4. Place veggies in large soup pot and cover with water.
5. Cook covered on low for one hour.
6. Strain.
7. Enjoy veggies as a side dish for dinner.

{preparation + cook time 1 hr **makes** 4 cups**}**

Conversion Chart

Volumes

US Fluid Oz	US	Imperial	Millitres	Dry Oz	Pounds	Grams
	1/2 teaspoon	1/2 teaspoon	2.5			
1/6	1 teaspoon	1 teaspoon	5			
1/4	2 teaspoons	1 dessert spoon	10	1		30
1/2	1 tablespoon	1 tablespoon	15	2		60
1	2 tablespoons	2 tablespoons	30	3		90
2	1/4 cup	4 tablespoons	60	3 1/2		105
4	1/2 cup		125	4	1/4	125
5		1/4 pint	150	5		150
6	3/4 cup		175	6		180
8	1 cup		250	8	1/2	250
9			275	9		280
10	1 1/4 cups	1/2 pint	300	12	3/4	360
12	1 1/2 cups		375	16	1	500
15		3/4 pint	450	18		560
16	2 cups		500	20	1 1/4	610
18	2 1/4 cups		550	24 1/2	1 1/2	720
20	2 1/2 cups	1 pint	600			
24	3 cups		750			

Quick Volumes

Pinch is less than 1/8 Teaspoon
1 metric Teaspoon – 5ml
1 metric Dessertspoon – 10ml
1 metric Tablespoon – 15ml
1 metric cup – 250ml
1000ml - 1 litre – 1 ¼ pints

Oven Temperatures

Weight

1 pound of flour - 3 ½
1 pound of sugar – 2
1 stick of butter is ¼

C	F	Oven
90	220	Very Cool
110	225	Cool
120	250	Cool
140	275	Cool - Moderate
150	300	Warm - Moderate
160	325	Medium
180	350	Moderate
190	375	Moderate - Hot
200	400	Fairly Hot
215	425	Hot
230	450	Very Hot
250	475	Very Hot
260	500	Very Hot

Volumes

cups
¼ cups
pound or 110 grams

Index